In celebration of

_____

Nightingale Pledge

I solemnly pledge myself before God and in the presence of this assembly to pass my life in purity and to practise my profession faithfully.

I shall abstain from whatever is deleterious and mischievous, and shall not take or knowingly administer any harmful drug.

I shall do all in my power to maintain and elevate the standard of my profession and will hold in confidence all personal matters committed to my keeping and all family affairs coming to my knowledge in the practice of my calling.

I shall be loyal to my work and devoted towards the welfare of those committed to my care.

Message

Best Wishes

Message

Best Wishes

Message

Best Wishes

Message

Best Wishes

Message _____

_____
_____
_____
_____
_____

Best Wishes _____

Message _____

_____
_____
_____
_____
_____

Best Wishes _____

Message

Best Wishes

Message

Best Wishes

Message _____

_____
_____
_____
_____
_____

Best Wishes _____

Message _____

_____
_____
_____
_____
_____

Best Wishes _____

Message

Best Wishes

Message

Best Wishes

Message

Best Wishes

Message

Best Wishes

Message

Best Wishes

Message

Best Wishes

Message

_____

_____

_____

_____

_____

Best Wishes _____

Message

_____

_____

_____

_____

_____

Best Wishes _____

Message

Best Wishes

Message

Best Wishes

Message

_____

_____

_____

_____

_____

Best Wishes _____

Message

_____

_____

_____

_____

_____

Best Wishes _____

Message

_____
_____
_____
_____
_____

Best Wishes _____

Message

_____
_____
_____
_____
_____

Best Wishes _____

Message

Best Wishes

Message

Best Wishes

Message

Best Wishes

Message

Best Wishes

Message

Best Wishes

Message

Best Wishes

Message

Best Wishes

Message

Best Wishes

Message _____

_____
_____
_____
_____
_____

Best Wishes _____

Message _____

_____
_____
_____
_____
_____

Best Wishes _____

Message

_____
_____
_____
_____
_____

Best Wishes _____

Message

_____
_____
_____
_____
_____

Best Wishes _____

Message

Best Wishes

Message

Best Wishes

Message

Best Wishes

Message

Best Wishes

Message _____

_____
_____
_____
_____
_____

Best Wishes _____

Message _____

_____
_____
_____
_____
_____

Best Wishes _____

Message

Best Wishes

Message

Best Wishes

Message

Best Wishes

Message

Best Wishes

Message _____

_____
_____
_____
_____
_____

Best Wishes _____

Message _____

_____
_____
_____
_____
_____

Best Wishes _____

Message

Best Wishes

Message

Best Wishes

Message _____
_____
_____
_____
_____
Best Wishes _____

Message _____
_____
_____
_____
_____
Best Wishes _____

Message

_____

_____

_____

_____

_____

Best Wishes _____

Message

_____

_____

_____

_____

_____

Best Wishes _____

Message

_____
_____
_____
_____
_____

Best Wishes _____

Message

_____
_____
_____
_____
_____

Best Wishes _____

Message

Best Wishes

Message

Best Wishes

Message _____

_____

_____

_____

_____

Best Wishes _____

Message _____

_____

_____

_____

_____

Best Wishes _____

Message

Best Wishes

Message

Best Wishes

Message

Best Wishes

Message

Best Wishes

Message

Best Wishes

Message

Best Wishes

Message

Best Wishes

Message

Best Wishes

Message _____
_____
_____
_____
_____
Best Wishes _____

Message _____
_____
_____
_____
_____
Best Wishes _____

Message

_____
_____
_____
_____
_____

Best Wishes _____

Message

_____
_____
_____
_____
_____

Best Wishes _____

Message

Best Wishes

Message

Best Wishes

Message

Best Wishes

Message

Best Wishes

Message

Best Wishes

Message

Best Wishes

Message _____

_____
_____
_____
_____

Best Wishes _____

Message _____

_____
_____
_____
_____

Best Wishes _____

Message

Best Wishes

Message

Best Wishes

Message

Best Wishes

Message

Best Wishes

Message

Best Wishes

Message

Best Wishes

Message

Best Wishes

Message

Best Wishes

Message

_____
_____
_____
_____
_____

Best Wishes _____

Message

_____
_____
_____
_____
_____

Best Wishes _____

Message

Best Wishes

Message

Best Wishes

Message

Best Wishes

Message

Best Wishes

Message

Best Wishes

Message

Best Wishes

www.ingramcontent.com/pod-product-compliance
Lightning Source LLC
Chambersburg PA
CBHW081011170526
45158CB00010B/3000